Understanding Your Body Alignment
Health and Longevity

D1668154

Understanding
Your Body Alignment
Health and Longevity

*A Practical "How to" Manual
for You and Your Body*

HARMON HATHAWAY

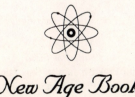

New Age Books

ISBN: 81-7822-001-6

First Edition: New Delhi 2000

First Published in 1996 under the title
"The Hathaway Alignment Sessions:
Alignment Discoveries for Health and Longevity"
by
Image Assembly V Press
Delhi, New York

© 1996 Harmon Hathaway

All rights reserved. No part of this publication may be reproduced
or transmitted in any form or by any means, electronic or mechanical, including
photocopying, recording, or by any information storage and retrieval system,
without permission in writing from the publishers.

Published by
NEW AGE BOOKS
A-44 Naraina Phase I
New Delhi-110 028 (INDIA)
Email: info@newagebooksindia.com
Website: www.newagebooksindia.com

For Sale in Asia Only

Printed in India
by Jainendra Prakash Jain at Shri Jainendra Press
A-45 Naraina Phase-I New Delhi-110 028

*This book is dedicated to
the memory of Monica Sonsia Lind Hathaway.
She has given us all a wealth of physical knowledge
that is the foundation of this work on alignment
and the roots of the first American Yoga.
Monica was a master of life's dance in space and time.
Blessed am I for having done the sacred pas de deux with her.*

TABLE OF CONTENTS

FOREWORD

BY DR. R.B. KELLEY SNODGRASS

The human body is a fascinating study. All the more so when the body we study is our own. As we learn about our bodies it is essential to have clear and accurate guidance. We are fortunate to have among us someone like Harmon Hathaway who has not only devoted a lifetime to the study of the body, but who is also capable of reporting to us what he has discovered. He is both an explorer and teacher. The book you hold in your hands is the gift of his knowledge. It is our challenge to mine the gems contained within.

Mining is different from shopping. The gems of this book are not necessarily laid out for us like jewelry in a shop. The work of active participation is required for us to realize the value of these lessons. This is a book we can read with our bodies. If you want to learn how to live within your body with more grace, efficiency, health and vitality, Harmon Hathaway's guidance can be invaluable. In working with Harmon over the years, I can personally attest to the validity, practicality and truth of what he has observed. I have incorporated many of these lessons into my personal life and into my professional practice working with patients , all with excellent results.

This century has seen some spectacular advances in knowledge about the human body, about its chemistry, physiology, genetics and pathology. But there is another area of knowledge which has been gaining increasing attention in the last fifty years, and that is the knowledge of how the body moves in space as an organized unit. At the beginning of this century we saw the development of the work of Methias Alexander whose study and insight led to the development of a system of knowledge now known as the Alexander Technique. Toward mid century we saw the development of Rolfing through the work of Ida Rolph with her emphasis on the muscles and related tissue in establishing what she called Structural Integration. About the same time we saw the emergence of the work of Moshe Feldenkrais who worked with the ideas of changing our mental structures by working with the Mind/Body interface, the

Feldenkrais Technique is the result of his years of research and teaching. Alexander Lowen was also at work at this time pushing forward the insights of the psychiatrist Wilhelm Reich into an psycho/physical discipline called Bio-energetics.

Since the 1960's, there has been a proliferation of methods and techniques which aim to solve physical (and mental) problems and optimize the use of the human body. The Hathaway Alignment Work, which has been evolving for over forty years, is now emerging at the end of this century as another step in the evolution of our understanding of the workings of the human body/mind.

The Hathaway Alignment Work shares with all of these body/mind disciplines, the requirement of conscious participation. The more we put this knowledge to use, the more we will benefit. Fortunately we have a capability of mind which we call "attention." One of the blessings of being human is our ability to direct our attention to whatever we will. Wherever we turn , the noise, bright light and sideshows of our carnival civilization compete for the attention of our eyes, ears, nose, organs of touch and taste. But when we close our eyes and turn our attention inward we make use of another sense, one which allows us to perceive the movement and position of our body in space. No less important than the other senses, it is often ignored and infrequently used in a deliberate and conscious way. I call your attention to this sense because it is an essential tool in working with this book. This sense has been given the name proprioception. It is the sense which allows us to know how many fingers we are holding up even though we are not looking at them. It is the sense which tells us if our elbow is bent or our head inclined or erect. It is a sense which can be developed and refined with conscious effort. Make conscious use of this sense as you work with the alignment sessions and other activities suggested in this book. Create the time and space you need to fully explore the depths of your body/mind awareness. Do this and you will be richly rewarded.

PREFACE

✧ This book provides an important step in our understanding of the human body by presenting a comprehensive view of Physical Alignment.

✧ Simply reading this book can bring positive physical results.

✧ The **Hathaway Alignment Sessions (HAS)** will be of great interest to practitioners of the healing arts as well as Doctors, Nurses, Chiropractors, Physical Therapists, psychologists and other health professionals.

✧ The knowledge of Alignment and Breathing may appear elementary, but, when experienced fully the results can be dramatic, powerful and lasting.

✧ Application of the discoveries in the book, **HAS,** cover the spectrum of health from severe illness to perfect health.

✧ The **HAS** can provide a direct and natural solution to many human illnesses, especially those related to: Emphysema, Asthma, Lung diseases, Bursitis, Tendonitis and Arthritis, to name but a few.

✧ The **Hathaway Alignment Work** can have a positive impact on problems such as Parkinsons, Cerebral Palsy, and Epilepsy, and in some cases achieve complete remission.

✧ The **Breathing** and **Alignment Sessions**, as delineated in this book, should be the foundation of early health education programs.

✧ Professional athletes can enhance their agility, stamina, grace, longevity and overall performance with the application of the **Alignment Sessions**. The retired athlete will find these **Alignment Sessions** important for releasing the tensions, stress and trauma that their respective sports have produced.

⬧ Many psychological problems become manageable and can diminish as a result of this work. The mental elements of fear and suffering can decrease as a result of becoming acquainted with the **HAS**.

⬧ Mastering what is presented in this book can enable you to understand many of the symptoms of your own physical problems and ascertain their solutions.

⬧ This knowledge is similar to discovering an element on the atomic chart. As such, any research in the fields of health using **HAS** can reveal new findings as well as provide a path to future insights of the human body.

⬧ For many of man's physical problems the **Hathaway Alignment Work** can indicate the cause, the remedy and a prescription for releasing these physical problems.

⬧ The **HAS** can reduce medical costs and health concerns for the business community, government and the general public.

⬧ The **Hathaway Alignment Work** provides fundamental data for the field of Ergonomics.

ACKNOWLEDGEMENTS

Thank you to the many friends of Monica and myself for the years of support and physical help in the development of this alignment work and the American Yoga Center, especially:

In USA, Bruce and Lori Lano, Geronimo Sands, Anne Joelle Lonigro, Gus Lightheart, Bala Pelletier, Marion Perkus, Cynthia Southmayd, Carolyn June, Michael Cook, Maggie Blair, Susan Rochmis, Fran Ciulla, Bill Stenz, Tamar Rogoff, Gillian Clements, Christopher Darsh, Jeffery Laudin, Fred Droshler, Stephen Stepka, Michael Kavorlavich, Edward Szydlik.

In Quebec, Maryse Pelletier, Jacques et Susan Danis, Marie Christine Jarrard, Nicole Chenut, Robert Boldac, Denise Corbeil, Janine Carreau, Charles Biname, and Claude Chamberlain.

Special thanks to Lori and Nicholas Swift of Image Assembly V Press for their help in the many drafts of preparation of this book. To Kelly Snodgrass for his technical assistance.

INTRODUCTION

A New Understanding

Alignment as defined in the dictionary means "to put in a line or line up." This will not do for a working knowledge that we can apply to the body. The primary concepts of alignment are of good posture or a straight back. This is vague and does not give us a knowledge that we can comfortably apply on a daily basis.

What you will learn in this book is that Alignment is not a static concept, but a dynamic principle of the body that you already have either active or in parts depending on your physical life condition. Fortunately, alignment appears as you work and learn more about breathing and releasing tensions.

This book was written to introduce you to the Hathaway Alignment Sessions, which can help you improve your overall health and performance by natural means. If you have current physical problems of any kind you may be able to find release from them by working with this book.

The Hathaway Alignment Sessions (HAS) are designed to help you release physical problems and restore your alignment. However, it is always advisable to get some medical opinion on problems of the body that persist and show no improvement. Use your common sense and experience when applying the sessions to your body.

The HAS were formulated, researched and applied by Harmon Hathaway and Monica Hathaway over 74 years of combined work experience in the field of physical counseling, therapy and yoga.

By understanding the principles of alignment you can have a new way of understanding the body in structure and function. This would be especially true in such fields as dance or athletics where performance is enhanced by correct alignment. You will also have tools for overcoming and understanding how to work with the many physical problems that life can present. By applying the principles of alignment and breath, you can have the ideal of a flexible, tuned and balanced body where motion is efficient, precise, effective and comfortable.

As a general plan for well being and natural health, the knowledge of alignment and breathing, as well as the other basics that are presented below, are invaluable for living healthy and longer. The sessions are low in impact and will result in physical releases, lightness, relaxation and discovery.

Chapter 1 presents alignment breathing principles for establishing and maintaining alignment. Once you have learned to breathe expansively and move with proper alignment, you are well on your way to experiencing the dignity and grace that are the natural elements of the body.

Chapter 2 on anatomy, acquaints you with the location of the body's joints, and describes how alignment helps the articulation of each joint. This chapter will show you how to bring greater flexibility to specific areas in your body by releasing tension in the joints that have accumulated through inaccurate use or incorrect ideas about a joints' location and articulation.

Chapter 3 will teach you about your body's capabilities for flexibility, balance and movement. The movement principles covered in this chapter will give you the experience of the body's potential for movement at the joints. You will also come to understand how to apply alignment while walking, sitting and standing. Again, the releasing of tensions and reduction of stress is part of the experience of this chapter.

Chapter 4 will provide you with Alignment Releasing Sessions to release the muscles and joints of the entire body. You can experience remarkable results after one session.

As you read this book, it is recommend that you also read this book with your body. There are many places in the book where you can spend time working with the principles of alignment. When that happens, allow your body to have the time to fully digest the principle or idea presented. There is no urgency to read on if you feel that you and your body are gaining a healthy insight from the text you are reading. Enjoy!

CHAPTER 1

*Bodily health is important, because it effects
our mental equanimity and concentration.*

BHAGAVAN SRI SATHYA SAI BABA

ALIGNMENT BREATHING PRINCIPLES

Knowledge of full breathing, or, using breath to develop and maintain alignment is not part of our general information systems. This chapter will fill this void.

To breathe is to live. If necessary, we could live for 40 days without food, for days without water, but only for a very few minutes without breath. If the brain is denied oxygen for only three minutes, serious deterioration sets in. Breathing is central to our very existence, and yet it is a process we tend to take for granted. We think of breathing as an "automatic" function our body will perform without our conscious attention, while we turn our minds to more important things. It is this *ignoring* of breath that is the cause of many of our physical difficulties. For infants, breathing is an automatic process. However, as we grow up, breathing is a process we can learn about and use in many different ways. For instance, when children in school are given a brief period of breathing instruction they will have a longer attention span and perform better.

You will discover in this chapter that there are many ways to use breath as a tool for correcting alignment, releasing tension, developing mental equanimity, improving your health and prolonging your life span. In this chapter we will first discuss the true role that breath plays in our lives. We will then present alignment breathing sessions that will acquaint you with the "tools" of breathing so that you may develop an "awareness" of breath and alignment.

Breath is the link between our bodies and the space of the physical world surrounding us. Through breathing there is a continual exchange between the inner and outer universe. The oxygen surrounding us is taken into the body to augment the building up and breaking down of molecules in every cell of our body. The carbon dioxide which we then exhale is used by green plants in the building up of their protoplasm that will then furnish us with food. The teacher, Gurdjieff, treated this transforming process of man and nature as an essential activity on the planet.

1

It is good to know that we can participate in life's essential processes by merely breathing.

Less widely recognized is the equally important function of breath as a link between the mind and the body. The breath of life provides a continual flow of energy, called *"prana"* by the ancients, that integrates the physical and mental aspects of the individual. Breath is intimately connected with thought and emotion. From the moment of birth, our breath is used to express our mental and emotional states. Through our speech and laughter, our sighs and cries, we use breath as a vehicle for psychic as well as physical renewal.

Unfortunately, a large part of what we call "growing up" is connected with our learning to control the way we express ourselves through our breath. We learn not to talk back, not to cry out with pain, not to laugh at the absurdities that we see, not to let our speech or tone betray uncertainty or anger. If we experience pain we are told not to "cry like a baby." We are told to "act like a grownup" and "don't make sound". We are conditioned to hold our childish and brazen impulses. We yield to the teachings of the adult world by, very literally, holding our breath. What we don't realize is that the unexpressed impulses don't go away, but remain as subtle tensions that accumulate within our bodies, showing up 30 or 40 years later as a major pain or internal problem. These difficulties can dissipate as you work with the Alignment Breathing Sessions.

Our body has an ability for absorbing what is accurate and useful. We should not underestimate this process but trust our body's ability to release and rejuvenate itself. Through conscious, full breathing we can reverse accumulated tensions that rob us of the structural grace that is our nature. By letting in a breath of fresh air—many breaths of fresh air— we can free the body and mind from the constraints we have imposed, and regain the freshness of the NOW that seemed lost.

So please, resist the temptation to understand the principles of alignment at once. As you work, you will start to grasp the meaning of these principles and feel the truth of them in your own body. First, discover how to open and relax the body, and then read and work with the various specific releasing sessions. Improvement will occur naturally.

KNOWING THE INSTRUMENTS OF YOUR RESPIRATORY SYSTEM

Before beginning a specific Alignment Breathing Session, let's try to see if we can understand what we are *not* doing regarding breath. It is helpful to have a sense of our present physical predicament.

Without changing your position, take note of how your body is positioned right now; You may be slouching in an armchair, or your upper body may be slumping over a table, chest collapsed down toward the stomach. This book may not be directly in front of you. You may be leaning forward into the pages, with your spine in an unnatural twist and your head propped up lopsidedly with one or both hands. Your legs, possibly, are crossed and held tightly together.

If you find you are in such a posture right now, do not change the posture, but attempt to take in a very full breath. I am sure you will feel the resistance or pressures that your breath has to push against to be full. As you work with the breath you will find that these collapsed, habitual types of bodily postures greatly inhibit the natural functioning and flow of the respiratory system. Likewise, the internal area of the body is asked to perform all its functions in a congested space. Generally, this is why we may feel tired and stressed at the end of a day.

Good News! The body is extremely resilient. As you start learning to work with the breath, years of poor postural habits and the subtle build-up of tensions can start to wash away. You will see and feel the differences as you perform the sessions. The accuracy of alignment and the increase of oxygen can have a dramatic effect on your entire being.

Through each of the following alignment breathing sessions, you can easily gain conscious awareness of breath. You will then be able to use breath to begin breaking up any ingrained mental and physical limitations you may have taken on.

THE STRUCTURE OF BREATH

The fundamental breathing muscle is the diaphragm, a large, dome-shaped, platform-like structure, horizontally bisecting the body beneath the lungs and heart. In the front, the highest part of the diaphragm connects just behind the bottom of the sternum (breast-bone). The diaphragm attaches in back to the spine and in front to the sternum. From these central points the diaphragm flows inward and slightly downward in all directions, connecting at the lower area of the ribcage onto and between the four pairs of flexible ribs.

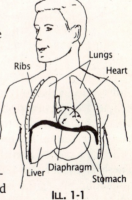

ILL. 1-1

Above the diaphragm are the lungs. Although we may think of the lungs as filling and emptying as we inhale and exhale, there should be some breath retained in the lungs after each exhale. We will refer to this

3

retention of breath as the "storage breath". The amount of oxygen you are able to retain in the lungs will increase as you work with the breathing sessions.

Similar to the technique of diaphragmatic breathing used by singers, this breathing will help you to maintain the structural integrity and alignment of the upper body. Your body should feel curved and full and rounded, not deflated. Deflating the lungs by exhaling all the breath can lead to physical and mental tiredness.

THE ELEMENTS OF FULL BREATHING

SESSION 1

Stand up in a space that affords you some arm room. Place your hands on your lower ribcage at the area of the flexible ribs, as in **Ill. 1-2**.

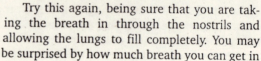

Now slowly inhale, taking a slow but full breath in through the nostrils. The chest will fill with oxygen and rise. Feel your flexible ribs expand with your hands. Slowly exhale and try to get the feeling of the breath rising and coming out of your mouth as you feel your lower ribs contract. The exhale will come up and out without the exaggerated use of the stomach muscles if you let your breath create the motion. The pattern feels as though there is a comfortable effort on the in-breath and a relaxation on the out-breath.

Try this again, being sure that you are taking the breath in through the nostrils and allowing the lungs to fill completely. You may be surprised by how much breath you can get in and retain in the lungs! Let the mouth open in a relaxed way. On this exhale, feel the breath creating the motion. When you have taken in a full breath and expanded the lungs fully, the air will exhale by itself, giving the impression of the breath rising and leaving by itself.

ILL. 1-2

The air comes into the nostrils just above the pallet, as in **Ill. 1-3**. There is no need to pull air upward into the nostrils. This method of inhalation tenses the body, producing a rigid feeling, particularly in the lower jaw, neck and head. The passage for air is not in the upper section of the nose but is directly behind the nostrils and only slightly upward.

When you inhale, feel that the internal passage of your nose is wide. The action of breathing in should feel *gentle*, yet strong and forceful.

4

With your hands on your flexible ribs, continue to inhale and exhale slowly, until you feel comfortable with the in-and-out action of the ribcage, and the flow of air into and out of the body. Be aware of how the actions of the breath fill out the three-dimensional space of the body, both inside and outside.

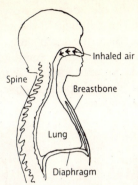
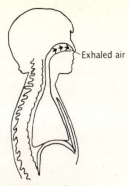

Inhaled air

Spine

Breastbone

Lung

Diaphragm

ILL. 1-3   BREATHING IN
As air is inhaled the
diaphragm moves down.

Exhaled air

BREATHING OUT
As air is exhaled the
diaphragm moves up.

Now place the thumb of one hand on the point where the diaphragm connects to the bottom of the sternum and the fingers of the other hand on the collarbone. Locate these points as in **Ill. 1-4**.

Slowly inhale, taking a full breath in through the nostrils. Fill the entire chest cavity and the abdomen. You will notice that the sternum and the collarbone between your thumb and your fingers go up. Slowly exhale, letting out about 1/3 of the inhaled breath from the stomach while keeping a "storage breath" in the upper chest cavity. Your upper lungs should stay full, and your sternum and collarbone should stay in place.

In diaphragmatic breathing you don't deflate the upper lungs when you exhale. If you experience a downward motion at the sternum or at the collarbone, you are letting out too much air and are deflating; you are not exhaling. Deflation causes the rib cage to collapse and the internal organs to become crowded and cramped. On the exhale, the upper ribcage maintains a storage breath; in deflation, the entire ribcage collapses downward. So keep working with this breathing process until you feel your collarbone retains the initial height that you had with your first inhale.

Breath travels into the lungs, then from the lungs, through the bloodstream, to every cell of the body. Each cell can freely rejuvenate itself with oxygen, ridding itself of waste products on the exhalation.

ILL. 1-4

5

As you breathe, *get the idea* that every organ and every cell in your body is breathing fully. This will help in the expansion of the upper body by not limiting the breath to the lungs. You will feel the action of the breath reaching up through your neck and down towards the legs. Every organ in your body has its own internal space. Your use of expansive breathing increases the internal space of your body, so your organs can function without being congested.

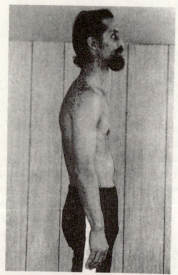

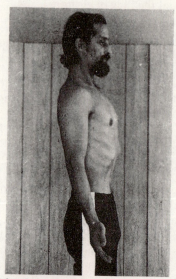

ILL. 1-5   DEFLATION   ILL. 1-6   EXHALATION

If you look at **Ill. 5 & 6**, you can see the difference between a true exhalation and deflation. As you can see, deflation is a falling and collapsing motion, while in an exhalation the position of the upper ribcage is sustained. The falling motion of the ribcage inhibits the interior space of the body and throws off your alignment. Breathe as fully as you can, making sure you are exhaling and not deflating. Continue breathing consciously, filling out the curves of the inner space of your body.

Many problems with the internal organs can be traced to the decrease of the upper body's internal space. This occurs when we allow the ribcage to collapse down, limiting our breathing to a shallow breath that hardly moves the ribcage. Full breathing increases the internal space of the body. Common sense tells us that if there is more space, then the whole metabolic process can function in a non-congested, flowing manner.

As you breathe fully, feel that the entire ribcage, back and front, including all its bones and the enclosed lungs, have a round three-dimensional

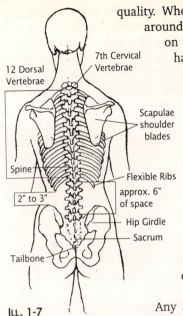

12 Dorsal Vertebrae

7th Cervical Vertebrae

Scapulae shoulder blades

Spine

2" to 3"

Flexible Ribs approx. 6" of space

Hip Girdle

Sacrum

Tailbone

ILL. 1-7

quality. When the ribcage expands, it expands all around, in the back as well as in the front and on the sides. Let go of any image you may have of a waist line; this allows the breath to fill out the lower abdomen.

You should keep playing with this familiarization of the pattern of diaphragmatic breathing until you feel you have an experiential understanding that you can take with you to the Alignment Releasing Sessions that follow.

The ribs—24 ribs, 12 on each side—are circling around the lungs. They connect at the sternum, (the breastbone), and circle around to attach to the twelve dorsal vertebrae on each side of the spine. See **Ill. 1-7**.

Like the ribcage, the spine is not straight. Any attempt to straighten the curves in the upper spine for "good posture" tends to pull the shoulder blades together and cause rigidity in the area of the neck, shoulder girdle and arms. The shoulder blades gently rest on the natural slope of the ribcage in the back. Any attempt to straighten the curves in the lower area, the lumbar, sacrum and the tailbone tie up your leg and hip motion. The natural line of the spine emerges as a result of releasing the bodies structural tensions which you can do by working with the Alignment Releasing Sessions.

When you breathe fully, you will notice that the shoulders get higher and rounder, thereby creating a spacious and restful platform for the head and neck to sit upon.

As you breathe fully, allow your attention to range over your whole body and note any areas that may feel tense and are not allowing the breath to expand into them. In the body there may be areas which harbor fear or self-consciousness, and these areas will have habitual tensions that stop breath from reaching them.

You will discover that it is possible to feel the action of the breath reaching down to your genitals and anus. It is possible breath will circulate in these areas once you have relaxed the mental-physical idea that you should keep this part of the body unresponsive.

The armpits are also an area of inhibition that we should learn to keep open. This generally comes from the nobel idea of not wanting to intrude

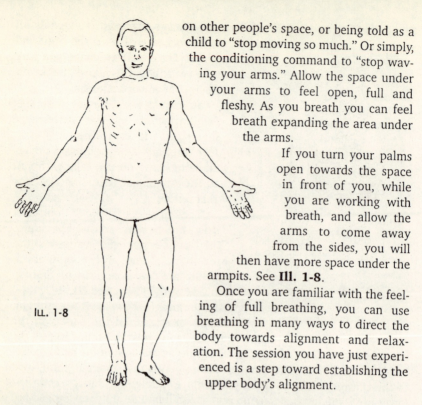

on other people's space, or being told as a child to "stop moving so much." Or simply, the conditioning command to "stop waving your arms." Allow the space under your arms to feel open, full and fleshy. As you breath you can feel breath expanding the area under the arms.

If you turn your palms open towards the space in front of you, while you are working with breath, and allow the arms to come away from the sides, you will then have more space under the armpits. See **Ill. 1-8**.

Once you are familiar with the feeling of full breathing, you can use breathing in many ways to direct the body towards alignment and relaxation. The session you have just experienced is a step toward establishing the upper body's alignment.

ILL. 1-8

USING BREATHING TO RESTORE ALIGNMENT AND HEALTH

AN EXPLANATION

When you are working with expansive breathing and you feel pains or aches in any area of the body, continue the breathing to help release the underlying pressures. Pains or aches are generally caused by a congestion or a collapse of the space in an area of the body, or from trauma caused by injury. So wherever you feel painful pressures, direct your awareness to the painful region and consciously bring the action of the breath to play in that area. Deliberately direct the inhalation and exhalation to that spot, with the intention of giving the organs and the systems flowing through the area more space in which to release.

You would feel claustrophobic in a very small room with no windows. This is also true of your individual cells. If the internal space of the body is cramped, then the cells also suffer from a lack of space and oxygen.

8

Similarly, you can feel hemmed in mentally by pressures from the external environment. Breathing will also help give you mental space in which to function.

When working with people who have physical problems, such as headaches, cramps, back pain, menstrual pains, soreness in muscles, etc. we have the client do deep breathing and direct the breath to the areas that have problems. The positive results are often dramatic. Breathing fully for expansion brings warmth and gentle activity to the affected area, allowing a renewal of the life forces. Breathing through emotional crises of various sorts also helps to alleviate the cramped, tense emotional state that may prevent you from seeing your way through the problem.

As you breathe life into a constricted area, you may feel an enlivening of sensations like tingling, numbness or pain in the area. This is because you are focusing your attention on the painful area as opposed to resisting the area. You are feeling what is already there *now*, and bringing the area to the foreground so it will be able to be processed and released.

It is important to allow any fear or other emotional reaction that arises to release itself. By focusing your attention on both the inhale and the exhale, fear or concern can be observed and allowed to pass. Should sound want to come out of the body, do not stifle it. Let whatever spontaneous feelings or sounds, such as "aaahh" or "oooww," that wants to emerge on the exhales, come out. Don't expect sounds to make sense to your rational mind. Simply allow your sounds to express themselves as you work with the breath.

Resistance to the sound or consciously stopping a sound that wants to come out of your body can cause additional body tension that would keep areas of the body closed off and entrapped with pressure. Resistance to pain or expression is counter-productive, and requires a great deal of energy. Allow discomfort, allow sound, allow that which wants to arise, occur, and pass away. Work on your painful areas consciously and gently. You can find the results very gratifying.

Whatever arises while you are working in an alignment breathing session is inevitably beneficial, and is an element of the body's releasing. The body will not hurt itself while working with breath, nor will the body present anything that you can not handle. Any somatic's like pain, trembling or shaking, that arise as you are working with breath are a result of the body's intelligence using the opportunity to release and free itself. **Your body is your friend. Trust it.**

A common sensation that appears in initial sessions for many people is a tingling and numbness in the hands and arms. This is fine. The oxygen is reaching the arms and hands via the blood stream. Eventually trembling will occur. This is very good since it is a releasing action that gives positive results when you persist. If a sensation like tingling or numbness persists after your session is over you can simply clap your hands, shake your arms, and normal sensations will return. Very likely, you will experience a freer more flexible feeling.

Besides your breathing having a healing effect on the organs of the body, full breathing brings about an improvement in the structural alignment of your body. As you become more familiar with using breathing as a tool for expansion and alignment, you will find muscles beginning to regain their natural length. The bones and joints release to their natural structural placements and your body will develop more flexibility. This becomes exemplified by the ease and fluidity of movement you will experience as your body releases. You will recognize the results whether lying down, sitting, standing, walking, dancing or running.

EXPANDING THE LUNG'S STORAGE CAPACITY

SESSION 2

In the previous session, we experienced the feeling of full, relaxed three-dimensional breathing into all areas of the body. In the following session we will consciously work to help our respiratory system acquire and maintain a full storage breath.

THE STORAGE BREATH AND PANT

Although our lungs have the potential to store up to three quarts of air and exchange up to four quarts in vigorous exercise, we tend to use about 1/4 of that storage capacity. Consequently, we run out of breath faster than we should. This session will help you experience the releasing dynamics that develop with full breathing.

Place a mat or blanket on the floor and lie down on your back. Place your arms slightly away from the torso with the palms of your hands facing up and open. Your chin should be drawn down toward the collar bone, as in **Ill. 1-9**.

Take a full deep breath in through the nose that lifts your ribcage up toward your chin. Allow your collar bone to rise upward with the breath.

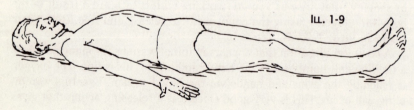

ILL. 1-9

It is alright if your shoulders rise up toward your ears as long as your shoulder blades don't pull together or become tense.

Next, exhale through the mouth about 1/4 of the air you inhaled. Make sure this exhalation comes from the abdominal area, and that your chest or upper body does not move downward. Inhale again, allowing your lower abdomen to expand as fully as possible. Let go of any ideas of having a waist line. Feel that your abdomen can have the expansive quality of a balloon. This will relax the abdominal muscles. As you inhale, let the action of the breath become so full that you experience an expansion throughout the entire stomach area, chest cavity, and up through the back of your neck.

You can breathe slowly, using a very gentle force. Draw the breath in, filling your body as full of oxygen as possible until you feel that the breath starts the exhalation without conscious effort. Then, exhale, letting out approximately 1/4 of the breath. Gently start to inhale again, repeating the process. While all this is going on, feel your mouth relax open, with a smile that brings the corners of your mouth towards the ears.

The breath that you are maintaining in the upper body is the "storage breath". It is this storage breath that helps develop the elements of alignment for the body and provides a way of maintaining the structural integrity of the upper body.

After taking the first breath in through your nose continue the full breathing in and out through the mouth. Inhale through your mouth and feel the width of the breath passage as the breath moves in and out. This is a panting breath. The image of a panting dog can be used here. While you are panting concentrate on the inhalation, using it to keep the body full of oxygen, the exhale happens as a result of being so full of oxygen.

Take in a full, deep breath that lifts your ribcage up and gives you a full rounded feeling in the upper body while also expanding the stomach region and lower back. When you exhale, only allow 1/4 of the breath to flow up from the abdomen and out through the mouth. Remember to maintain the storage breath in the upper chest cavity. If any of the storage breath has dissipated, add more breath. Keep inhaling and exhaling slowly, through your mouth. Repeat this panting action, checking to make sure that you are maintaining the structural alignment of the upper body and have not lost any of your storage breath.

As you pant, notice that your flexible ribs move in and out at the sides of the body and that there is a similar motion of expansion and contraction in the muscular space between the ribs. If this does not seem to be happening, it means that you are losing some of the storage breath. To keep the storage breath from diminishing, only concentrate on the in breath of the pant. If necessary put your hands on your ribcage or

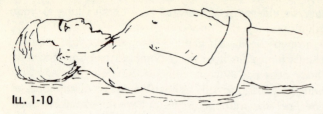

ILL. 1-10

abdomen as in **Ill. 1-10** until you are certain your body has accepted the pattern.

Do this panting with a full storage breath for as long as is comfortably possible. If your mouth becomes dry, breathe through your nostrils for a while and then return to the mouth. As you continue the pant, you may notice a slight trembling in the back or chest. This is a good sign, indicating that the breath is expanding into areas that had formerly been dormant or bound with muscular tension.

You should resist any temptation to stop. Just slow down and feel the breath as it enters and leaves your body. Continue to work with the breath and trust the natural intelligence of your body to use it. As you do this for longer periods, you may also experience tingling or a numbing along the arms and even across the lower jaw and lips. This is a releasing function of the body and is a good sign. The tingling and numb feelings are very common when first starting to work with the panting breath and nothing to be concerned about. This indicates that the releasing activity is starting. As you continue to breathe, releasing will start in your upper body and could reach down through the hips and into the legs.

This session should be done for at least fifteen minutes at first, and then for longer periods as you become comfortable with this breathing action. This breathing exercise will also acquaint you with some of the body releases that you will have in your upper body. Generally there is an expansion of the rib cage that remains after the session is over and a feeling of being taller and lighter.

This session is a good way for you to recover after strenuous exercise or activity. You can do the panting breath while maintaining the fullness of the upper body when you are running or walking. It should be noted that panting is not "the way" to breathe all the time, but a way of using breath as a tool for releasing and establishing alignment.

FULL BREATHING WITH THE STORAGE BREATH

SESSION 3

In this session you will work with keeping the storage breath full while breathing in and out. The idea is for you to work with the momentum that builds over 20 minutes as you are keeping your body expanded. Your body can have a sequence of releases—one after the other—that peels off layers of resistance to expansion.

Lie down as in the previous exercise and take in a full storage breath. Inhale and exhale slowly through your nose, letting out as much air as you can on the exhalation without losing your storage breath. Breathe slowly with the idea of allowing the breath to fill your whole body. Imagine the breath expanding out into the space around your body. Do full breathing with the idea of giving the breath to your body to utilize however it wishes. Trust the intelligence of your body to release whatever hidden tensions you have unconsciously been harboring, and to fill out and expand any cramped muscle groups or skeletal collapses that have occurred. When you finish this breathing session you will experience increased energy and relaxation.

As you are working with this full breathing you may experience trembling and shaking in various muscles groups throughout the body. This is a releasing action of muscles that have been "held" and are subsequently tense. These muscles are now "unwinding", giving the body a softer, fuller, more flexible feeling.

This low impact, Alignment Breathing Session should become the foundation of one's knowledge for releasing and restoring the body's health and well-being.

When asked "how long should I do this session?" I will remind the client; "You can't over-breathe."

BREATH AND SOUND

SESSION 4

The following session will enable you to be conscious of breathing while producing sounds. Many people seem to lose the sense of the breath when they speak or produce sound. In a conversation you may not only hold your breath while speaking, but may also hold your breath while listening, since you are busy focusing your attention on listening and being polite. As you grow to understand breathing in your every day life you will be able to listen or speak and have space for breathing at the same time.

This session is also useful in familiarizing you with the dynamics of sound and how sound can help in the releasing of tension from your body. Our natural tendency would be to express the sound that any event warrants, whether the sound is a soft sigh from tiredness, or a loud sound of joy. However, we are conditioned out of expressing sound in so many ways, both subtle and not so subtle, that we hold the impulse to make sounds which requires a freezing of many groups of muscles.

Very often babies will make loud or odd sounds, but before the sound can be fully explored an anxious parent may arrive with a bottle or a "pampering" interruption. This conditioning continues through childhood whether it is at home or in school. We are all familiar with how loud a child can speak in the supermarket or library and the parental need to make their child be quieter. However, let's not blame the past for our limitations but use the *present* to experience what sounds are possible.

Lie down on your back, arms out, palms up. Take seven full breaths in and out. On the eighth breath exhale slowly, whispering a pure "aah" sound (not "eeh" or "ugh"). Keep your mouth open, with the jaw relaxed down and open toward the collar bone. Vary the opening of your mouth to find a position that does not interfere with the sound. Experiment until you find a comfortable tone.

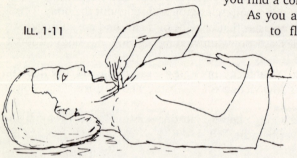

ILL. 1-11

As you are allowing the air to flow out from the abdomen, check to make sure you have not lost your storage breath. As in **Ill. 1-11**, you may want to place one hand on your collarbone and the other on your abdomen. This will help you to feel the air releasing completely from the abdomen without losing the storage breath. You should have the feeling that the sound is traveling up and out on the breath and not being pushed out by the abdominal muscles

As you are working with the "aah" sound, you can let the volume of the sound increase by stages after every eighth breath until you are making a nice large sound.

The "aah" sound should fill your mouth and resonate through the throat. You may also feel the sound vibrating in the chest cavity. You can feel the coolness of the breath touching the insides of your throat and mouth and you can feel how wide the passage for air is.

Let the sound of "aah" fill the room without evaluating the quality of the sound. Simply let it occur. Throughout the session, be sure your sound is coming out directly from your mouth, rather than having a nasal sound.

After you have gotten comfortable with the varying intensities of "aah", experiment with "haa". The "haa", unlike the "aah", will come up in a single, burst on the rapid exhale. Place your palms on your abdomen and feel the upward movement of breath as you let out a powerful "haa". Now experiment with "hoo" and "ha, ha, ha, ho". Feel as though the breath is making the motion of exhalation rather than the muscles of the abdomen.

As you practice these sounds, you may experiment with new sounds or even words and sentences. The idea is to get the sensation of the sound riding on the breath. Thus, when you speak, your words flow outward with the breath, and are not being pushed out, interrupting the natural rhythm of breathing.

This session is very exploratory, and you may find many different sounds that you like to make. This will be releasing for you and very relaxing. The vibrations that resonate in your throat and chest are like an internal massage.

When you are having a conversation you can practice spacing your words with breath. It is an interesting exercise and will retain energy rather then dissipate energy. For public speakers and actors this practice is very rewarding because of the character it can give to your performance.

FREEING THE JAW, THROAT AND FACE WITH BREATH AND SOUND

SESSION 5

In this session, we will consciously attempt to free the areas of the jaw, face and throat. You may feel silly as you do the session, since it will require you to "make faces", as is often seen with children. Don't worry about these feelings. Just allow them to come and go without thinking about how you look or sound. You may do this session standing, sitting, or lying down.

Allow your mouth to relax open while drawing in a comfortable, full breath. Let your tongue relax and come out of your mouth, resting on the lower lip. As you are taking an easy in and out breath through the mouth, move the corners of the mouth up towards your ears with a big smile. Then relax your mouth back to the original position. Repeat this for a minute or so expanding and contracting the facial muscles. The breath should feel very wide as it passes in and out of the mouth and throat.

Now start to move the muscles of the face and head as you are breathing comfortably. This is exploratory and will help you become aware of all the muscles of the face and head. Play with this for a while as you are comfortably breathing.

Now you can start an "aah" sound, and let it drift out of your mouth on each exhale. Remember to maintain some storage breath in the upper lungs throughout this session. Next, alternately increase and lower the volume of the sound you are making so that it has a sing-song quality. When this is comfortable and interesting to you, you can then try to move the quality of the sound up and down, from very nasal to deep in the throat. This will give you a full range of possibilities of sound to play with.

As you are making sounds let the sounds change tone and volume. This can be done in a stream of consciousness style where you let the sound change by itself. If you can match the sounds with changes in facial expressions that would also be interesting and releasing. While experimenting in this session you may also find that you have some physical releases, as well as losing some inhibitions.

Summary

The Hathaway Alignment Breathing Sessions that you have done should become a part of your daily or weekly program for relaxation and rejuvenation. As you progress you should select the sessions that work for you and give you the best results.

Using expansive breathing is very important in your everyday life for maintaining Alignment and physical health. As you work with expansive breathing your body will become fuller and more aligned. The breathing will become easier, the results more evident, as you progress.

In all your activities - standing, sitting, walking, dancing and running, talking and singing, reading, writing and playing at a computer, be aware of the living space of your body. Remember to consciously feed your body the nutriment it thrives on, the BREATH OF LIFE.

CHAPTER 2

In the beginning was the creation,
and forever after, the maintenance.

BRUCE LANO

MAKING FRIENDS WITH YOUR SKELETON

In working with a variety of people, I have found that surprisingly few people can visualize how their own skeleton is constructed, the exact location of each joint and what range of movement is possible at each joint. This lack of accurate knowledge of one's own skeleton can cause undue muscular tensions that inhibit flexibility and balance in any activity. If you have an inaccurate or vague idea of how your body moves at each joint, this inaccuracy or vagueness becomes translated into your motion. We then develop a style to handle the imbalances, like the walk of John Wayne, or the body movements of Richard Nixon.

When you have felt alignment and understand where the joints are located and how the bones move at each joint location, the body's potential range of motion will expand. This can be a dynamic process that involves your instinctual movements which are precise and efficient.

As you acquire an accurate view of how your bones and joints connect, you will be able to feel the joints' origination points. This understanding is essential when you are working to achieve alignment. In other words, if you are moving with an erroneous or vague idea of where the articulation of bones and joints are, you can create tensions and compound problems.

ILL. 2-1

In this chapter you will have a chance to experience your skeleton, joint by joint. As you come to know your body better, it will become increasingly clear which areas need the most release and relaxation. You

17

can then work with the specific Alignment Releasing Sessions in the other chapters to address your specific needs.

As you work with the simple movements in this chapter, don't force the joint action by using the large muscle groups to move your foot or hand. Leave your muscles relaxed with as much of a "fleshy" feeling as possible. You will see that movement originates with your intention to move, and not in the joint or muscle itself.

Understanding that the intention to move comes before movement is a subtle fact. An example that you can feel is: lifting an arm up over your head by intending to put your hand over your head. This movement uses muscles with less effort then if you were to lift the arm over your head while the hand remains limp. In professional dancing and sports this subtle difference can be very important during performance.

THE JOINT

At the joint, bones are tipped with cartilage, a smooth material that is softer than bone, which cushions the joint. This is enclosed by a thin membrane (Joint capsule) which contains Synovial fluid and provides a smooth surface for articulation of the joints.

ILL. 2-2   DIAGRAM OF A TYPICAL MOVABLE JOINT

This system of cartilage and synovial fluid lubricates and prevents wear and tear on the joint.

When your muscles become tense, the space at the joint becomes compressed. In extreme cases of tension, the membrane can become damaged and cartilage can wear down. Prolonged muscular tension can cause joint pains of various types and degrees. Many problems arise in the joints because we don't know what alignment is. This results in pressures that are contrary to the proper use of the joint. We must learn about alignment to release tensions and to create a sense of space for movement around and in the joints of the body.

Each joint allows for the independent movement of a part of the body, yet because of muscular tension and imbalances in the body we may find that we are unable to move one part of the body without another part becoming tense or wanting to move also. Each leg, for example, has a free swing space of its own, but as we raise one leg, the other tends to react as well. Relaxation through the joints will help alleviate these conditions, allowing a greater range of movement.

The movements in this chapter are designed to help you experience the location and potential motion in the major joints of your body. In the Hathaway Alignment Seminars we start by giving this informal type of introduction on the skeleton. I have been told, afterward, by doctors, nurses and other health care professionals, that they enjoyed the hands-on experience of knowing the skeleton through examining their own body. Some professionals admitted to having an erroneous view about the location of a joint. The study of anatomy should be a hands-on experience that locates all the joints of the body in addition to a clinical examination of a chart.

Later, in the individual sections and especially in the final section, you will find specific Alignment Releasing Sessions designed to release muscular tension in the joints. However, before you begin to make specific corrections in the body, you should know the bodies movement potential at each joint as well as the alignment design that nature intended.

Perform the movements in this chapter to improve your understanding of your body. Through your understanding of this chapter on the skeleton (which presents very important yet very basic information) you will come to appreciate the alignment and breathing sessions and how they release your body to alignment as they are freeing up your joints.

THE FOOT

Each foot is composed of twenty six bones and twenty six joints allowing for tremendous flexibility and movement. We should be aware of the fleshy, flexible quality of the foot which can be as nimble as the hand.

Stand up and feel the weight of your body moving down the legs into the ground through the outside pad of each foot. Now slowly raise your toes and lower them one at a time, little toes first. If you don't experience the movement of each toe individually that's OK start where you are. Play with this movement of the toes.

ILL. 2-3

Standing with feet pointing straight forward, press into the ground with the outside pads of the feet, allowing your heels to raise until you are standing on the ball and toes of each foot. As you are moving up and down you can feel that by pushing down against the ground the body lifts up.

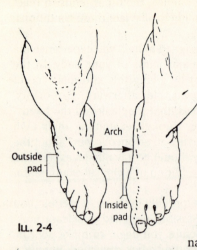

Arch

Outside pad

Inside pad

ILL. 2-4

You don't lift the body, you use the ground, a subtle and interesting feeling.

Make sure the weight is dropping into the ground primarily through the outside pad of the foot so the arch of your foot keeps a natural curve. Relax your knees and feel that your legs are not locked. Now let's try this by pressing from the inside pad of the foot. You will notice that when you press the ground down using the inside pad of the foot, the body tends to lean forward and your balance is narrowed to a thin line up the center of the body. This throws the body's alignment off. Another interesting and subtle point, but the very root of your alignment. You will come to appreciate that a properly aligned body begins with the feet.

Ill. 2-4 shows outside pad and arch.

In standing, the arch of each foot is maintained by focusing your attention on letting the weight move into the ground along the outside of the feet. This is fundamental for correct body alignment. This principle of alignment will be treated more extensively in the standing and walking sessions.

THE ANKLE

Most people have an erroneous idea about the location of this joint, imagining it to be higher than it is. The ankle joint is located at the end of the lower leg beneath the two lower leg bones (tibia and fibula) where they meet with the bones of the foot.

Using your hands, locate the inside and the outside process of the tibia and fibula. Feel the points where they connect with your foot. Move the foot while your hands are holding the ankle. You can feel all around the ankle to locate the source of motion as you are moving your foot.

Sit down on a chair or on the floor and raise one foot at a time. Rotate the foot first toward the

ILL. 2-5

Tibia

Fibula

Points of articulation

outside, and then toward the inside, so that you feel the movement in the ankle. Now flex your foot upward toward your shin, and then extend your foot downward as far as you can as in **Ill. 2-6**. Repeat, using the other foot. Simple repetition of these motions and rotating your foot will help acquaint you with the range of movement in the ankle.

ILL. 2-6

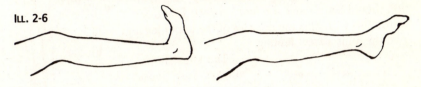

THE KNEE

The knee joint joins the lower leg bone (tibia) and the upper leg bone (femur). The knee joint is actually below and behind the knee cap.

When you bend the knee to kneel down, the patella (knee cap) slides down to provide a pad for the surface at the end of the upper leg bone. You can find the joint location at the inside and outside of each leg. The knee cap is easy to feel but, the location of the knee joint is harder to find. Move the lower leg while you are locating this joint.

Kneel down and move the lower right leg up towards the buttock. Lower the right leg, and perform the same motion with the left leg. Now you can feel that when you are on your knees, the knee joints are still free to move. Contact with the ground is being made by the knee cap or patella, just like a pad for you to kneel on.

Standing on your right foot, raise the left foot up and then swing the left foot straight out (Ill. 2-9). Put your attention on the back of your knee joint and feel the source of the movement. Now swing in slow motion. Repeat the swing, standing on the left foot. We can feel that the

ILL. 2-7

Femur
Patella or knee cap
Tibia
Fibula

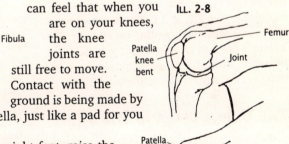

ILL. 2-8

Femur
Patella knee bent
Joint

Patella
Tibia
Joint

21

movement of the knee originates at the back of the joint. Generally we tend to put the weight of our body down through the front, inside part of the knee. This puts an undue strain on the joint, and throws the body forward and off balance.

While you are moving the lower leg, the intention should be to move the foot backwards and forward. This will relax the muscles of the upper leg and give the joint a freer feeling.

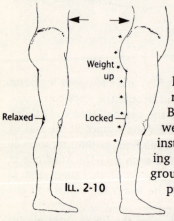

The knee should always feel "loose" as opposed to "locked" when you are standing. See **Ill. 2-10**. The habit of locking the knees is probably responsible for leg and lower back problems that develop as a result of many years of standing this way. By locking the legs we tend to pull the weight of the body "up" out of the ground, instead of allowing the ground we are standing on to receive the weight of the body. The ground supports the weight of body. The pulling of the weight "up" out of the ground creates imbalances and counter balances which cause stress.

The habit of placing our weight on one leg or the other when we are standing can put tension on the hip sockets where the upper leg bones join the hip girdle. See **Ill. 2-11**. The habit of locking your knees and standing on one leg at a time is not bad or wrong, but you should be aware of how you are standing, so you don't create tensions over the whole day.

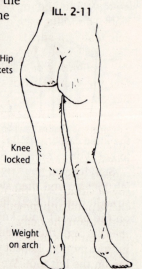

THE UPPER LEG AND HIP JOINT

The hip girdle is composed of the two large bones (Ileum), that have joint connections at the sacrum and in front at the pelvis. The articulation of these joints are not really discernible, but we should think of the hips as two bones, rather than a solid bone that goes all around the body.

22

During pregnancy the tissue of the joint at the pubic area softens and becomes flexible to create space for birth. The image of the hip girdle being a cradle for the baby to rest in is a good way of viewing a function of the hip girdle. In pregnancy, the baby will be carried in the hip girdle, if you are creating space by breathing fully and have correct alignment.

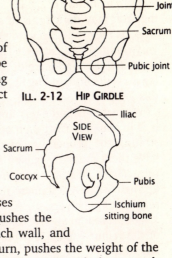

ILL. 2-12 HIP GIRDLE

The hip girdle is a region where many people's alignment problems originate. From very early in life many people have a tendency to tuck the genitals back, either from early toilet training anxiety or from negative sexual conditioning. This causes a lift of the tailbone and sacrum, which pushes the lower intestines forward against the stomach wall, and causes an inward turn in the legs. This, in turn, pushes the weight of the body toward the arch of the foot, which is not in touch with the ground. Later in life this "tucking", which has become habitual, shows up in fallen arches, knee trouble and lower back problems as well as possible internal problems.

The hip girdle also provides a house for the lower organs to sit in. Ideally, your lower organs should not be lying against the stomach wall. This will create a protrusion of the stomach wall (paunch). Many of the Alignment Sessions for the legs are designed to reverse the tendencies of turning the legs inward and the tucking in of the pubic bone. See **Ill. 2-13**.

ILL. 2-13

In doing Hathaway Alignment Sessions you can feel the body release to a natural, aligned position where you can feel that your weight is shifting to the outside of the feet and your hips have the feeling of sitting with the weight dropping towards the ground. Alignment is a result of releasing, not a concept that you place upon the body.

If you look at the skeleton (**Ill. 2-14**), you will notice that the upper leg bone connects to the hip girdle higher than imagined. It is a common misconception to picture the legs beginning on a line with the crotch. This

23

idea inhibits the full swing of the leg, and leads to a limiting of the leg swing in walking. You may notice this in some people, who, as they walk, seem to shuffle with a very limited leg swing. This is easily remedied by understanding where the leg joins the hips and feeling the motion of this joint.

When I encounter this limited use of the legs in clients, I start their session by demonstrating the proper use of the leg joints and have them practice walking for about ten minutes. That's all it takes for most people to free up their walk. A testament to the human bodies rejuvenating powers.

Let's stand up and try to find the outer process of the femur [upper leg] bone with your hands. **Ill. 2-15**.

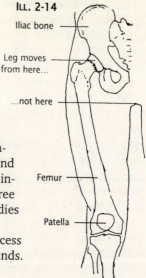

ILL. 2-14
Iliac bone
Leg moves from here...
...not here
Femur
Patella

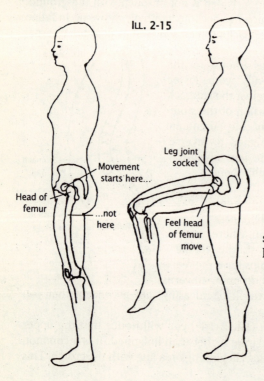

ILL. 2-15

Movement starts here...
Head of femur
...not here
Leg joint socket
Feel head of femur move

While feeling this bone, bend forward from the hip joint (not the waist or crotch) without your buttocks moving backward, as in **Ill. 2-16**.

Run your hands along your buttock and hamstring muscles and try to let go of any tension so the muscles feel as soft as possible. Then slowly rise and stand upright. Experiment with this bend several times, while your hands feel the joint and muscles involved.

Start a walk, very slowly, with your hands feeling the outer process of the upper leg bones. Feel the action of the leg joint as you walk around so you are aware of the height of this connection at the hip girdle. The length of your stride and how high you can lift your leg in towards the body, all illustrate the use of this joint.

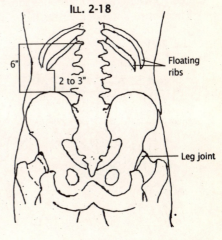

ILL. 2-16

THE SPINE

As you can see from the illustration of the spine, the lower back is composed of the coccyx, the sacrum and lumbar portions of the spine. The sacrum and coccyx consist of fused vertebrae. The motion in the spine begins at the first joint of the lumbar section and continues upward at each vertebra. See **ILL 2-17**

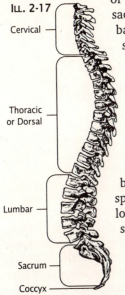

ILL. 2-17

Cervical

Thoracic or Dorsal

Lumbar

Sacrum

Coccyx

There should be about six inches of space in the back lumbar region from the top of the hip girdle (sacrum) to your first flexible rib and approximately two to three inches on the sides. See **Ill. 2-18**. If the muscles in this area are tight, the space becomes compacted. Generally the shortness of the space between the ribs and the hips is a result of shallow breathing. Even in bodies with a lot of weight the skeleton is actually thin. The breathing sessions will expand this area open.

ILL. 2-18

6"

2 to 3"

Floating ribs

Leg joint

The upper spine is composed of the twelve dorsal vertebrae to which the ribs attach. Then the seven cervical vertebrae above which complete the spine.

SESSION 1

To experience the full flexibility of the entire spine, this movement is excellent. Lie down on your back with your knees bent

25

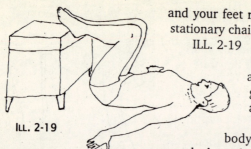

ILL. 2-19

and your feet resting against the seat of a stationary chair or couch as in **Ill. 2-19**.

ILL. 2-19

Now press against the chair and lift the buttocks off the ground until you feel a full arch in the back (**Ill. 2-20**).

Let the weight of your body move down into the ground through the neck and shoulders.

Slowly lower your body feeling it touching the ground vertebra by vertebra. Repeat this motion several times and relax any tensions that prevent the movement from being smooth. This particular movement is good to do occasionally just to loosen up the vertebra of the spine. Generally 4 or 5 times is sufficient.

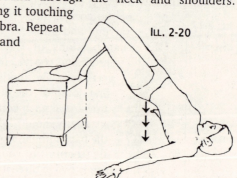

ILL. 2-20

THE SHOULDER GIRDLE AND THE ARMS

The shoulder girdle is composed of the two collarbones (clavicle). two shoulder blades (scapula) and two upper arm bones (humerus). This interlocking structure has only one skeletal connection with the trunk of the body, where the collarbones join the top of the sternum. **Ill. 2-21**.

The entire shoulder girdle has a free-floating nature that allows for extensive movement and flexibility. If you trace the collarbone out, with your fingers, from the top of the sternum to the shoulder, you can feel where it joins the top of the scapula above the shoulder joint. The humerus (arm bone) joins the underside of the scapula to form the shoulder joint.

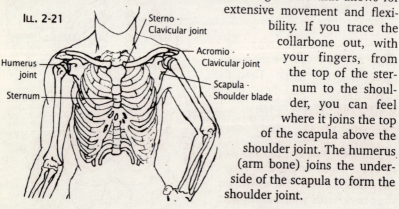

ILL. 2-21

Sterno - Clavicular joint

Acromio - Clavicular joint

Humerus joint

Scapula - Shoulder blade

Sternum

ILL. 2-22

The following movements will allow you to feel the full flexibility of the upper body.

ILL. 2-23

Lift the shoulders up toward the ears and then bring the shoulder blades together, as in **Ill. 2-22**.

From this position, lower the shoulders and then raise them again. Now open the shoulder blades and bring the shoulders forward and then lower them as in **Ill. 2-23**.

Repeat the same sequence of movements with the arms raised straight above the head as in **Ill. 2-24**.

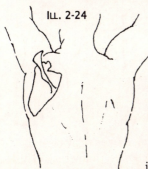

ILL. 2-24

SESSION 2

The shoulder girdle becomes limited because we haven't understood the free floating nature of the three part joint system. Your collar bone is the only bone connected to the rest of your skeleton, the rest of the bones are connected with muscle. Later in this book you will find alignment releasing techniques that help release the muscles that cause stiffness and prevent full movement.

ILL. 2-25

Many people suffer from one of two conditions: either the muscles of the shoulders are strained away from the spine in a forward hunch, or they are jammed toward the spine in a militaristic posture. Both conditions are unnatural and lead to many aches and pains.

The upper arms' joint is not at the top of the shoulder but underneath it. You can experience this by placing the fingers of the left hand an inch below the top of your right shoulder, while swinging the right arm from the joint below. Repeat with the opposite hand and shoulder. See **Ill. 2-25**.

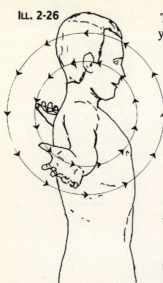

ILL. 2-26

The following movement is designed to help you feel the whole rotation of the shoulders and arm joints. See **Ill. 2-26**.

Raise your hands straight out to the sides, palms up and rotate your arms backward tracing four small circles. Then four medium-sized circles and finally trace four large circles. When you start this movement focus your attention on the hands initiating the movements. This will help you to relax the larger muscles of the back and arms. If you are having joint problems at the shoulder, work very easy with this motion, keeping the palms and hands open. This movement reverses the closed rotation that the arms tend to be held in, which builds up an abrasive use of the shoulder joint. See **Ill. 2-27**.

ILL. 2-27

Turn in

Side View

Back View

THE ELBOW AND WRIST

The elbow is a three-point connection joining the upper arm bone (humerus) with the lower arm bones (radius and ulna). You can experience two types of motion at the elbow: flexing and extending plus a rotation of the lower arm. Experience the rotation by keeping the upper arm still and turning the palm up and down. See **Ill. 2-28**.

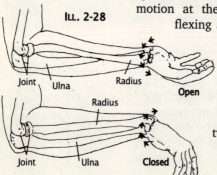

ILL. 2-28

Joint   Ulna   Radius   **Open**

Radius

Joint   Ulna   **Closed**

The wrist is composed of the two lower arm bones and three bones (carpels) in the hand, which allows for extensive motion. See **Ill. 2-29**.

THE HAND

The hand alone has 27 bones and 27 joints, which enable people to perform such incredible feats of flexibility and speed as playing the piano, castanets, guitar and typing.

ILL. 2-29

SESSION 3

Walk around and allow the hands to relax open with the palms facing forward. Let the fingers open so that you can feel the air passing between each finger. If you feel that the fingers want to move allow them to move. If your fingers remain motionless, then intentionally start them moving. Your fingers and hands should take over the motion in time.

Ulna

Radius

Wrist joint

Explore all the types of motion that you can get when you relax the hands and fingers. You may feel that they want to shake and move very actively — go with it! In many cultures the hands and fingers are very expressive and play an important part of ceremonies and dance. We also see this in many styles of kung fu.

THE HEAD AND NECK

Above the 12 dorsal vertebrae are seven cervical vertebrae, which make up the neck. The sixth vertebra, the axis, allows the head to rotate from left to right, while the seventh, the atlas, allows the head to move up and down. **Ill. 2-30**. The combined action of the atlas and axis allows the head to make a smooth, rotary motion.

When we turn our head left and right, up an down, the movement originates at the atlas and the axis. We can feel this by focusing our attention on these vertebra. Many people are inclined to move the

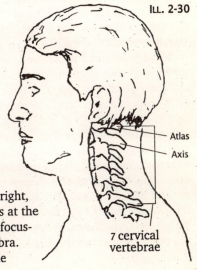

ILL. 2-30

Atlas

Axis

7 cervical vertebrae

29

head with little awareness of this origination point. The attention is on the jaw and face, causing the face and head to protrude forward which makes the body lean forward slightly as we are turning our head. **Ill. 2-31**. Understanding this alignment principle is very important for feeling the alignment of the upper body. **Ill. 2-32**. In performance this principle is especially important if you are performing a series of ballet turns, diving, or doing gymnastics.

If you straighten the back of your neck in the area where the atlas and the axis are and let the jaw rest close to the collar bone you can KEY the alignment of your upper body. As you make this shift of the head you can feel the rib cage rise up and the breath come in to fill the space you have just created for the lungs.

ILL. 2-31

The following movements will help you feel the head turn while your attention is on the exact location of articulation.

Take a full storage breath and relax the chin toward the collarbone. Then slowly turn your head to the right until your chin is over your shoulder. Get the feeling that you are moving from the back of the head. Repeat this slow turning of the head from shoulder to shoulder about 10 times.

Move your head all around, up and down with your attention on the cervical vertebra, which is the origin of the motion.

In summation, each of the movements in this chapter will aid you in locating and moving accurately from the principal joints in the body. You should be able to extend what you have learned about your body from this chapter into various activities. You will appreciate this chapter more as you work with the Breathing and Alignment Sessions in the other chapters of this book.

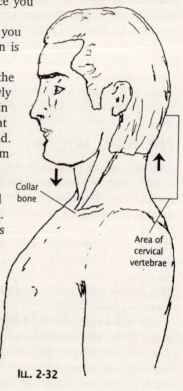

Collar bone

Area of cervical vertebrae

ILL. 2-32

CHAPTER 3

It was mindfulness on respiration
that acted as the basis for the seeker to attain enlightenment.

NARADA MAHA THERA

BALANCE AND ALIGNMENT

When our body and mind are in conflict we experience a loss of health and vitality. Many people impose an idea of how they should look onto their bodies, which cause distortions of posture and muscular tension. A typical example is the way some men and women walk. The strong macho stride of the male is as common as the slinky, seductive walk of a female. Both, of course, are unnatural and eventually cause stress and tensions, as well as internal problems. The male and female bodies already portray their natural sexuality. Exaggerated efforts to emphasize a gender or cultural ideal only masks the body's true nature.

People who want to get ahead in the world, or who are always running around in a rush, do so with their heads and shoulders leaning forward into the space in front of the body, leading with the head (instead of with the feet). The action of walking becomes one of the muscles of the body struggling to maintain their balance.

Many physical problems are inherited because of a lack of information about the bodies alignment. We bring subtle distortions with us from childhood, whether from our parents postural habits, the admiration of a fictional hero of the movies, or a body type we choose to imitate.

Fear, which is as common in the western world as aggression and ambition, can cause the body to become tense in a subconscious retreat from the world. Life has become so fast-paced and success oriented that it is rare to find anyone without undue muscular tension. This misuse of energy deprives us of vitality and stamina.

If we are moving our bodies without the efficiency of alignment, tensions become compounded. Ideas about "winning" and "getting ahead" make the situation worse because the body is constantly being "conditioned" from an aggressive point of view. The idea of winning is inherent in every game, but our awareness should be on the activity itself—not the outcome. An open body that is aligned and structurally balanced will be able to master action as it occurs.

The sequence of sessions in this chapter are designed to help us let go of tensions that distort our balance and posture as we discover the correct

31

principles of alignment while standing, walking, jumping, running and sitting.

Session 1

Using the Full Ground

There is an old saying; "you have to be able to crawl before you can walk." In this session you are going to crawl, to experience the flexibility of your back muscles as you used them as a baby. You are going to become reacquainted with the use of the body while on all fours. This is also effective in "freeing up" stiff torso muscles and rigid mental views. As you are moving around allow yourself to feel like a child or an adolescent.

This session is easy to do and playful so let your body "play" with the movement and enjoy itself. Choose a room with as much uncluttered space as possible, preferably with a well–cushioned rug or mat on the floor.

Get down on your hands and knees in the center of your work space and drop the lumbar region of your back down toward the belly button area.

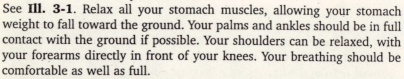

See **Ill. 3-1**. Relax all your stomach muscles, allowing your stomach weight to fall toward the ground. Your palms and ankles should be in full contact with the ground if possible. Your shoulders can be relaxed, with your forearms directly in front of your knees. Your breathing should be comfortable as well as full.

Slowly, crawl in a straight line using opposite hand from knee. Crawl to the end of the room and then back again. Do this crawl four to six times and then crawl in a large circle around the room. Once you have gotten a comfortable feeling with crawling, try crawling at different speeds. Turn around in one spot or make longer crawling strides. As you play with this movement, you may feel like a baby or an animal. A baby crawls without knowing the word crawl. At the baby stage, we were all free to "discover" movement, rather than imitate the movements of others.

Ill. 3-2

Now feel the movement of a cat. Make long, slow reaches with the hands and knees as a cat does when it stalks its prey. Feel the gentle strength of the spine, and the grace that the cat puts into each

32

move. Feel any tense areas and try to relax them so your movements flow like a cat.

The cat, like the baby, is a master of natural movement. The ability to move naturally with the body relaxed, on your hands and knees is within you. This session will help you to rediscover that feeling. See **Ill. 3-2**.

SESSION 2
THE BASIC STANCE

We all can learn more about standing. The simple act of letting the ground support the body is a surrender we are unfamiliar with. In the martial arts being grounded is the root from which all action flows. When your body is out of alignment you are resisting gravity. In this session you will learn how to let your weight settle into the ground and release tensions.

We spend most of our waking hours standing. We can use this time to release tension or stress instead of taking it to dinner. By applying the principles of alignment to the stance you also start releasing tensions that currently exist in the body. You may have been holding tensions in the legs for years yet, when you start standing in alignment your body can start to release tensions.

Lets start by locating, in our own stance, some of the common tendencies that contradict alignment and then we will correct them.

Stand up with the weight of the body on both legs and look down at your feet, ankles, and knees. If you notice that your legs have an inward turn that causes the legs to lock and lets the weight of the body move down into the ground through the arches of the feet, you have what is generally considered a normal stance.

What we usually call a flat foot or a fallen arch is an extreme example of the common tendency for the weight of the body to shift onto the insides of the feet and legs. Even if you have a high arch, you may still notice an inward turn at the ankle. See **Ill. 3-3**

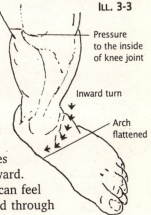

ILL. 3-3

Pressure to the inside of knee joint

Inward turn

Arch flattened

If your knees are locked and your thighs have an inward turn (See **Ill. 3-4**) then your pubic bone will be rotated under and back toward the buttocks, causing muscular tension in the lumbar region of the spine. This forces the upper body forward and the muscles have to adjust to keep you from moving forward. If the conditions described above exist, you can feel the weight of the body going into the ground through

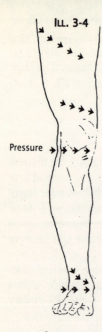

ILL. 3-4

Pressure →

Weight drops down

ILL. 3-6

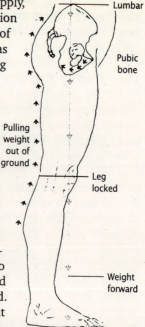

ILL. 3-5

Lumbar

Pubic bone

Pulling weight out of ground

Leg locked

Weight forward

the front of the feet instead of the whole foot, See **Ill. 3-5**. If none of the above seems to apply, that's good. Doing this session will give you a clear feeling of what alignment is as well as produce some interesting releases.

Stand with your feet about 6 to 8 inches apart and your feet facing straight ahead. Roll outward from the bottom of your feet, so the majority of your weight goes into the ground through the outside edge of each foot. You can exaggerate this turn-out because it reverses the tendency to roll the weight to the inside. Your knees should have a slight bend and be relaxed. Let your hip girdle shift so that you have a feeling of sitting, allowing the weight to drop and move down and around the legs into the feet and ground. Get the idea of the weight rotating out from the inside of each leg to the outside, so that the weight settles into the ground along the outside edges of the feet, chiefly under the anklebone. **Ill. 3-6.**

Start doing deep breathing that lifts the upper body and maintains the storage breath. This raises the rib cage so that you have the full space between the ribs and the hip girdle. Continue this full breathing throughout the session.

Bring your chin in towards the collarbone as you continue to breathe. Let your arms be comfortably at your sides and face your palms forward with the fingers separated and straight.

Bend your knees slightly and relax the muscles of your lower back, allowing the tail bone to settle down with the feeling of sitting. This will cause the genitals

34

and front of the pelvis to gravitate forward and upward. When you find the right position, you should feel that your body is standing directly over the ground you are on.

You may feel the leg muscles start to vibrate right away. If not, as you stand in this position for ten minutes or longer you will start to feel a slight tremble in the muscles of the legs. This is a "releasing" action. Welcome it. You can facilitate this releasing action by bending your legs at the knees and then straightening them. This bend should be minimal, just enough to get the trembling action started. The idea here is for you to play with and encourage the trembling that begins as you are standing.

As you work with your stance you may find that the legs want to go into other movement. Allow this action. It is very important to allow your body to do what it wants to do. The movements are the "unraveling" of tension from your muscles. Trust your body while you are experiencing the movements and the subsequent releases.

Try to do this basic stance with full breathing for about twenty minutes. If your feet start to feel uncomfortable, take a few steps in place and continue the session. You will have considerable insight about your body from this experience. You will learn how to listen to your body. You will learn how the body wants to move and release.

You should try to do this basic stance once a day until you feel that the activity of vibrating and releasing is out of your legs. The basic stance is useful when you are involved in a sport that requires a lot of running. Try doing the basic stance during the pauses in the activity. This will keep your legs from tiring. If you watch professional runners you will notice that they often stand with the legs shaking off or moving to loosen up the muscles of the legs. This shaking off movement is what you may encounter, as well as the trembling, while you are doing the basic stance.

If you have problems with the legs, knees or feet, you will find that working with this session is very helpful. You should try to do a session of 20 minutes of standing 2 times a week. You can reduce this as you feel the legs releasing. There are times when you can take the position of the basic stance from 2 to 5 minutes and have a release of tension that you may have been accumulating. There are times in everyone's day when the basic stance can be applied in an informal manner.

SESSION 3
WALKING

Learning to walk while you are maintaining alignment is interesting and useful. We may not have given too much consideration to our walking, assuming that we have managed well enough so far. Let's start by saying that walking is an art that has had many uses in history. There is the samurai that is ever present and grounded, with feet that glide across the ground. The hunters of many cultures were trained to feel every step as they moved.

In the 20th century the importance of being aware of the ground and your interaction with the ground is confined to sports and gymnastics. We are in need of some accurate alignment information regarding walking and running. The following session will give you the basis for establishing alignment while walking.

Stand in the basic stance, leaning slightly backwards into the space behind the body, so your weight is towards the heels. Take a full storage breath raising the rib cage. Allow your weight to settle into the ground through the heels, along the outsides of the feet, and extend your hands about 12 inches from the sides of your body with your palms facing forward and your fingers separated and extended.

In slow motion, lift one foot placing it down heel first, one step ahead, without taking the weight off your back leg. The leading foot is just touching the ground with no feeling of weight in it. Slowly begin to shift your weight to the foot in front, simultaneously moving the back foot upward and forward. Keep your attention on the sole of the foot and place it down heel first, one step ahead. Again, the weight remains on the back leg and foot. Repeat this walk in slow motion so you can feel the feet leading in the walk. The feeling is that you are walking from the space in back of the body.

Make sure that your knees are relaxed. If the knees feel tense, allow them to bend slightly throughout the movements. Be sure to move from the sole and not the tops of the feet, which keeps the ankles relaxed. Also check to make sure you are stepping with the weight on the outside of your feet.

The emphasis here is to land the foot that leads in the walk without putting any weight into it. Then as the weight shifts into it, the other leg will swing forward with ease. Again, land without putting any weight into this step until you are ready to move. **Ill. 3-7.**

As you develop a rhythm in this slow–motion walk, there should be no feeling of using your muscles deliberately

ILL. 3-7

Weight on back foot

to lift and move your foot upward and forward. The mere intention of moving will start your muscles moving in a natural way. There should be no strain in your legs. The back foot that remains in line with the ground should not tense up or participate in any way as you move the opposite leg forward. Let each leg move in its own space.

As you are moving, experience a feeling of leaning slightly backward into the space behind the body. Be aware of the back of the knee joint and get the idea of walking forward from the space behind you. Walk slowly in a large circle until you have a full, comfortable awareness of your movement. Then increase your pace and complete three to four circles around the space.

To increase your pace, simply speed up the rhythm of the movement for a full minute, then increase the speed a little more for another minute until you are walking fast. Your attention is on your feet leading in the walk while your upper body is being carried forward. If you watch a little child who is just starting to walk you will generally see what has just been described in action.

Once you are comfortable with a normal walking pace, you should again slow down and make sure you have the feeling of walking forward with the feet leading, not the upper body.

Session 4

After you have become comfortable walking in this fashion you should allow a period of about 20 minutes to introduce a variation, described below, that will help in releasing the body while walking.

In this variation you will work with the principle of giving the body's weight to the ground. This is accomplished by taking shorter steps and allowing the feet to land with all the weight of the leg going into the ground. You can hear each step as it lands and makes a definite sound. You might even exaggerate the force of the foot landing, as if you are marching. As you do this you can feel the muscles of the legs and buttocks relax and bounce. Being truly grounded is what you are accomplishing when you apply alignment and give your weight to the ground.

This variation of walking and giving your weight to the ground should be done for ten minutes at first, until you can feel the difference between walking and holding the weight in the body and walking while you give the weight of your body to the ground.

Session 5

Allow 20 minutes for this session. You will be taking your body for a walk and permitting your body to show you how your body would like to play with the walk.

You begin by walking, as you have just learned, with the weight of your body being given to the ground. As you are walking around your space, allow your body to change the walk or present what it feels like doing. You do not have to think about this, just keep moving at a steady pace and your walk will change. Your body may start marching or walk with the feet slapping the ground or take short steps and stomp the ground etc, as we see little children do. You are allowing your body's intelligence to present what it has to do to release and unwind the muscles that have been conditioned or held in a stylized way.

You will find that taking long walks and working with the alignment breathing is easy to do and establishes good physical alignment habits.

Applying the alignment principles when running is important since problems resulting from incorrect alignment are compounded when running. Correct alignment when running will result in a more efficient runner. One key to apply is using the outside of the feet, which helps to maintain the arch of the foot. If you have knee or hip problems this will help reduce the problem because you are compounding alignment. This is an area that you can explore for some very interesting results.

The breathing sessions and working with the storage breath while you are running will help you find what is useful for you to extend your stamina and increase your speed. Keep a diary-the discoveries you make are worth sharing.

SITTING

Sitting is a position we are finding ourselves in more and more as the work environments change. If you do much sitting at work it is an excellent opportunity to apply alignment to the body. If you are not sitting with a knowledge of alignment and

ILL. 3-8

ILL. 3-9

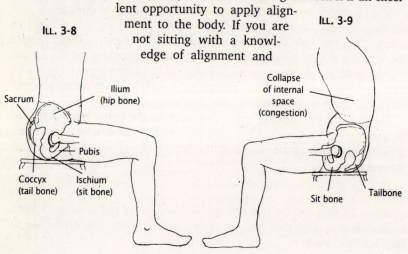

Sacrum

Ilium
(hip bone)

Pubis

Coccyx
(tail bone)

Ischium
(sit bone)

Collapse
of internal
space
(congestion)

Sit bone

Tailbone

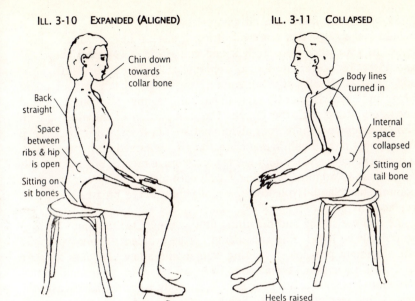

ILL. 3-10 EXPANDED (ALIGNED)

Chin down towards collar bone

Back straight

Space between ribs & hip is open

Sitting on sit bones

Feet on floor

ILL. 3-11 COLLAPSED

Body lines turned in

Internal space collapsed

Sitting on tail bone

Heels raised

breathing you may be subject to general tiredness, where you find that you are constantly moving around trying to find a position that is relaxing. The most common complaint that **people** have is of progressive back, hip or leg problems which they blame on sitting all day.

The key to sitting is knowing were the sit-bones are located and utilizing them. By sitting on the sit-bones you will bring correct alignment to the sitting position. If you look at **Ill. 3-8 & 3-9**, you can see the difference between sitting on your sitting bones and sitting on your tail bone.

In **Ill. 3-10**, the feet are apart, the spine straight but not rigid. The neck is straight and in line with the shoulders, while the lower jaw is relaxed down toward the collar bone. In this position the body will not tire and can be rejuvenated with comfortable full breathing. Your body is kept erect by your skeletal position and your breathing maintains proper alignment.

SESSION 6

Allow about 20 minutes for this session. Sit on a bench or hard chair with both your feet firmly on the floor and the weight of the legs dropping into the ground along the outsides of the feet. Be aware of the seat beneath you, and make sure you are sitting on your "sit" bones and not on the sacrum or tail bone. As you are sitting, move back and forth and side to side over the sitting bones. This can have the quality of a baby rocking in a chair.

39

Sit with your hands placed comfortably on your thighs. Your spine should feel straight but not rigid. Bring your chin in towards the collar bone, so your neck feels straight and your head is centered above the shoulders. The lower jaw should feel loose and relaxed. **Ill. 3-10**.

Now start to take in a full comfortable breath that fills your upper lungs and expands your rib cage. Inhale fully feeling your collarbone and shoulders lifting with the breath. The last portion of this deep breath should reach down into your abdominal area in front and in back. Keep breathing. Do the diaphragmatic breathing as described in chapter 1, with a panting action and without losing your storage breath. Breathe like this for at least 10 minutes, allowing your breath to become slower and more comfortable. Should you lose some of your storage breath, be sure to replace it.

As you are sitting and breathing fully you may feel like moving your feet and legs. This is fine and should not be avoided. As you work with the alignment principles of sitting, you should allow your legs to move and have their play. Again, your body will start to move and release stored up energy that has been held in the body. Explore and discover-the results that you have are your barometer.

As a discipline I suggest that you apply what you have learned about sitting while taking a long trip in a car or train.

SUMMARY

The standing, walking and sitting sessions that you have done, should be done often. The insights that you get about your body's alignment are progressive. All three sessions are basic body activities that you can apply to your daily life. By becoming aware of your body's alignment in your daily life and maintaining the integrity of your body's structure you can maintain good health and feel more relaxed.

CHAPTER 4

The future waits, the present demands action.

"ANTIGONE" — SOPHOCLES

ALIGNMENT RELEASING SESSIONS

Physical alignment can become subdued or hidden by the way a person treats and regards the body. If you work out with the idea of conditioning the body by tightening the muscles of the body, rather than opening, loosening, and discovering your body, you create tension in the joints by shortening the distance between the areas that the muscles lay across. An example of this is the sit-up. This exercise tightens the muscles of the stomach wall (abdominal) and creates less space internally as well as shortening the distance between the hip girdle and the rib cage. The reason that most people do a sit-up is to get a flat look to their stomach. You will accomplish this by expanding the body open and having the length of the muscles of the stomach. An aligned body is healthier and gives you the appearance you want.

The efforts to build muscles of "steel" and have a body that looks "good" can limit the flexibility of the body. An aligned and released body truly looks good. This may be different for the professional athlete who follows a specific program for his or her sport. Although, the athletes also need to understand the principles of alignment and releasing. For the general public the preference should be to have flexibility and alignment.

Many people's ideas of relaxation means, allowing their body to become limp and collapsing on a couch or chair instead of releasing the tensions that consume their energy. If we are to uncover the structural integrity of the body, we need to examine the ideas of relaxation, strength and flexibility as they apply to our activities, and our body.

Relaxation is an active principle that we administer to the body. The basic misconception that prevails is that relaxation is a moment when we are inactive. This misconception is counter productive since it leads to a disposition—physical, mental, emotional—which closes down areas of the body. Our breathing becomes shallow while our body postures tend to contract. This causes stress by the reduction of the internal space of our body. It also creates subtle tensions in the muscles of the body because we are holding the breath still. Gentle expansion with breath is more relaxing for the body then a static contraction. You will understand this as you work with the releasing sessions below.

Strength, as an idea, needs to be studied more thoroughly in the West. For the context of this book we shall just suggest that a flexible strength is the ideal most of us are looking for. It is the strength that we see in animals—a power of intention—rather then a strength that requires hours of lifting weights or conditioning.

Generally, the strength that develops doing physical work or playing a sport is fun and provides us with the opportunity to keep our muscles toned. Many people, like farmers or carpenters, have physical occupations that keep the body in shape. For those people who have a more sedentary lifestyle, they must find the time and opportunity to get physical. I suggest that to tone your muscles you find a physical activity or sport that you like and can have fun doing.

In relationship to alignment and learning the dynamics of breathing, the natural strength of our body should be sufficient. If however, one wishes to develop a specific strength for a competitive activity, you will find that your body will acquire the strength from spending more time doing the activity that is fun, then giving that time to working out and building muscles you think you need. When you are using alignment and breathing the natural strength that you have will appear. You then will recognize a type of strength that is proficient and powerful.

Flexibility already exists in the body's muscles and joints. If we lose flexibility as we grow up it is generally from misinformation, or the absence of accurate information about our body. When you don't have an idea of what alignment is and spend most of your life moving about in ways that are counter to alignment, the flexibility of the body becomes limited. We become aware of the loss of flexibility and attribute this to our age. Not so—you will experience the increase of flexibility as you spend time with the releasing sessions below.

You will understand that expansion and alignment are what give you true relaxation. Working with the knowledge of alignment will give you the tools to release tensions that currently exist, as well as preventing tensions and stress from building up. You can look forward to restoring the body to a greater state of relaxation, flexibility and strength.

The Alignment Releasing Sessions are designed to allow the action of "trembling" and "shaking" in tense muscles. Releasing the muscle knots will leave the body with a softer, fuller, more flexible feeling. Unlike regular stretching exercises, there is no application of force to expand the muscles. There is also no problem of muscles "snapping back" and having to be stretched again since the releasing of muscles restore the muscles to there intended length. The sessions may seem more time-consuming than regular stretching exercises, but in the long run they are more efficient, of low impact and the results are progressively deeper and lasting.

As you release tension from the muscles of your body you will be uncovering the physical alignment that was always there. Alignment is a result, not an idea that we put on the body.

If you have been working regularly with the basic breathing and alignment sessions presented in the previous chapters, you should already feel a change in your body. The body should feel fuller, taller, and more spacious. On the other hand, you may still notice areas in the body that feel tight and in need of releasing. There may also be tensions existing in the body that you are not aware of. The releases and the freedom of an area of the body after working with the sessions in this chapter often are beyond what we think of as feeling released. The Alignment Releasing Sessions in this chapter are designed to further your progress in achieving alignment by releasing entire areas of the body.

When you begin to work with the alignment releasing techniques provided in this chapter, you should have the idea of "intending" each movement, while applying the instructions for each movement. When it is suggested that you lift your foot off the ground this is different than suggesting you lift your leg off the ground, although to someone watching, the two different ways of lifting might appear identical. The real difference involves the muscles you use. An example is; if you intend to lift the foot in the air, you will use less energy and muscle then when you intend to lift the leg.

You should start each movement by following the directions given, until you have had a good period of release. Then you may explore the area of movement to see if you can uncover different areas that will give you releasing activity. You will discover areas where the vibrations intensify. This is what you are looking for. Do not try to control the body, and don't become concerned if the vibrations become very active or you feel like letting out any sounds. Use the exercises as a starting point, and then go with the spontaneity of the body. The trembling and shaking will cease when you end the session, at which time you will experience the results of your good efforts.

FREEING THE BODY

The sessions can bring greater flexibility to various joints, and will also speed recovery to an injured part of the body. Take your time with each session, working with each session as time allows. If you do the first session and get some good releasing, be happy with that and try another session when you can comfortably give it the time you deserve.

Twenty minutes is the recommended minimum for each session. If you work for thirty minutes to a full hour, you will develop a momentum that produces marvelous results.

Releasing the Pelvic Girdle and Thighs

Session 1

Muscular tension in the pelvic area is a big problem to the body, because it throws out the entire posture of the upper body. The space of the thighs and legs also become cramped.

ILL. 4-1

Releasing the pelvic girdle can make a dramatic difference throughout the body, while the resulting releases from a 1/2 hours work should give you the feeling of being more open in the legs and pelvic area.

The session requires a space were you can lie down comfortably while you put your feet up on a soft chair that will not move, or on a couch with soft cushions for your feet to set against.

Lie on your back, place your feet on the edge of a chair or couch so your knees are bent at approximately the same angle as in **Ill. 4-1**. Feel a firm pressure through the outside of your legs and feet going into the edge of the chair.

Slowly separate your knees by rolling both feet open until your legs are as open as is comfortable, without strain. Slowly bring the knees together by rolling the feet back to the original position **Ill. 4-2**. Repeat the same opening and closing movement for the period of the session. The opening of the legs should be faster then the closing of the legs. If you can, allow the legs to fall open and then bring the legs together very slowly.

An important feeling to have as you are doing this movement is; when you bring your legs together, *relax* the *inside muscles* of the legs and *push* the legs together with the *outside muscles* of the legs. It helps develop the releasing action if you are not pulling the legs together. This little shift of attention will produce excellent results.

Relax inside muscles

Push closed with outside muscles

ILL. 4-2

Continue to open and close your legs in this manner for at least 15 minutes. In time, shaking will occur in the muscles of the thighs and throughout the groin and pelvic area; it may even extend into the lower back. If you find one place in the movement where the shaking is greatest, confine your motion (slow opening and closing) to that area and explore the shaking to release tensions.

After your initial experience with the session, try doing this session for a longer period of time. You should make the judgement based on your age and physical condition. Again, the body will not present anything you can not handle when you are working to release the body. You can trust your friend, the body. Ideally a 30 minute session is good.

When you are finished with this session, start walking around your space and feel the body. You may feel a change in the way your body walks since you have had some releasing of the muscle groups of the legs and hips. Perhaps you can feel how the body is allowing the weight to go into the ground along the outside of the legs and feet, or you might sense that your body feels straighter. "Alignment is starting to appear!"

SESSION 2 ✕

This session is a variation of the session above. The pleasant element of this position is that you can do this movement anywhere that you can lie down on a firm surface.

Lie on your back with your knees bent and your feet flat on the floor, (**Ill. 4-3** and **Ill. 4-4**) about 6 inches apart and about 10 inches from your buttocks. Take a gentle full storage breath and continue to breathe comfortably and fully throughout the session. Extend your arms comfortably out from the body with your palms facing up and your fingers separated and extended.

ILL. 4-3

As you open and close the legs it is important you feel that you are closing the legs with the muscles of the "outside" of your thighs and relaxing the internal leg muscles, so you are not pulling your legs together, but, pushing them together with the outside muscles.

ILL. 4-4

The surface of the floor should not be slippery for your leg position to be stable. Your feet should be in contact with the ground with the weight going into the ground through the outside pads of the feet and the arch being maintained.

Allow the legs to come open, then bring the legs together slowly, letting the knees touch. Repeat this motion. You will start

45

to feel activity in the muscles of the legs after a period. When the muscles show a good amount of vibration, confine the movement of opening and closing to this area. Explore the area of vibration to see if you can find spots that increase the trembling.

After you have become familiar with both of the above sessions, you will find that you can go to an area where there was trembling previously and find some more activity. Then you can open and close your legs in that area for continued release. If you do not find any activity go back to the original movement of full opening and closing.

RELEASING THE KNEES AND THIGHS

The next three sessions will give you additional tools for releasing the lower body.

Lie on your back with two or three firm pillows under your buttocks so your pelvis is angled upward. Two couch cushions work well. Lower your chin so that it moves toward your collarbone and straightens the spine in the back of the neck. Extend your arms to the sides, palms up. Lift your feet off the ground until they are perpendicular to the ground. Without altering the position of the thighs or pelvis, slowly lower the feet, bringing the heels down towards the buttocks, as in **Ill. 4-5**.

ILL. 4-5

Concentrate on the movement of the feet and imagine them to be the source of the motion. Now slowly raise the feet, extending them again to the upright position without altering the position of the pelvis. There should be a feeling of pushing the air up with the foot as you raise and straighten the legs. Repeat this simple up-and-down movement and allow whatever trembling or shaking that arises to occur. Make sure your stomach muscles are relaxed during the course of this exercise.

Eventually you will feel a shaking in the legs, through the pelvis, and along your lower spine. The more intense the shaking is, the greater the release of pent-up energies will be. We have found, when doing this movement, that there is usually one area of movement where the shaking is greatest. When you find this area, confine the up-and-down motion to it and allow the shaking to travel throughout your body.

This simple movement is effective for releasing different muscle groups of your legs, hips and back. You should do this session for at least 20 minutes.

VARIATION #1

This is a session that will reach different muscle groups of the legs and thighs. Lie on your back, with a firm pillow or two under your buttocks so that your pelvis is angled upward. Lower your chin so that it comes close to your collarbone, and extend your arms comfortably out from the sides of your body.

Bring your legs up until both legs are perpendicular to the ground and your feet are above the hip joint, with your legs straight. If you find it difficult to straighten the knee, place more pillows under the buttocks so you can get your legs to be straight. Slowly move the feet apart to get as large a "V" shape as possible without straining the groin muscles. Then bring the feet slowly back together until they touch. **Ill. 4-6**. Do this session for about 10 minutes.

VARIATION #2

This is another movement session to bring release in the pelvic area. Place a pillow under your buttocks and raise the feet until the legs are perpendicular to the floor. Slowly bring the knees down toward the chest, as far as they will go without forcing them, as in **Ill. 4-7**. Then slowly return to the original position with knees straight and legs and feet pointing straight up in the air. Repeat this movement for at least 20 minutes, allowing shaking to occur.

ILL. 4-7

RELEASING THE UPPER BODY

The next two sessions are wonderful for relaxing and releasing your upper body. This will make breathing fuller and easier. The sessions can be done for twenty minutes to an hour for maximum benefit. After you have a series of good releases from working in these sessions, you will find doing a session for five to ten minutes will relax you after a hard days work or play.

SESSION 3

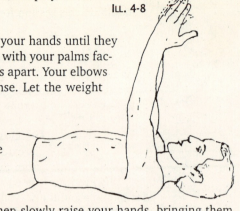

ILL. 4-8

Lie on your back and raise your hands until they are perpendicular to the floor, with your palms facing one another about 6 inches apart. Your elbows should be straight but not tense. Let the weight of your arms drop through your shoulders and into the ground so your shoulder blades are resting on the ground. Slowly lower your hands to the sides until they touch the ground and form a "T" with your body. Then slowly raise your hands, bringing them up until your palms meet. The intention is to move your hands up and down so you are relaxing your upper arm muscles. Move your hands and arms slower as they come up to meet. Breathe fully and comfortably during the session. See **Ill. 4-8** and **Ill. 4-9**.

As you do the many repetitions of your arms moving up and down you will start to feel a tremble across your chest and shoulders, which will eventually reach into your back. This, again, is the start of a releasing action. Allow the activity to occur. In some cases the shaking can even reach to your stomach muscles, that's fine, this means you will get some dramatic releases in your upper body. If the tremble is minimal, keep working and more activity will appear.

ILL. 4-9

SESSION 4

This session will release the muscles of the back along the spine as well as the rib cage.

Lie on your back and stretch your hands above your head, arms softly outstretched and palms facing each other. Bring your hands up slowly to a position over your head on a line with your eyes, then return your hands to their original position above your head. The moving of your arms down can be faster than when you raise the arms. Repeat this

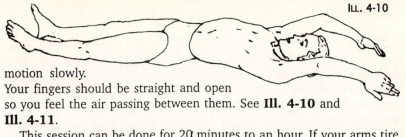

motion slowly.
Your fingers should be straight and open
so you feel the air passing between them. See **Ill. 4-10** and
Ill. 4-11.

This session can be done for 20 minutes to an hour. If your arms tire,
rest them for awhile and then continue the session. You will
find that the releasing action from this position can
become vigorous throughout your upper body. The pre-
liminary releasing can be substantial. After a few sessions the releasing will settle down.

ILL. 4-11

SESSION 5

Place a long pillow or two couch pillows on the ground. Lie down on
your back with your shoulders and head touching the ground and your
arms comfortably out as in **Ill. 4-12**. The rest of your body should be up
on the cushions including your feet. Move your arms up slowly to a ver-
tical position. Now start the arms down toward the ground as in Session
4. Repeat this motion for the duration of the session,

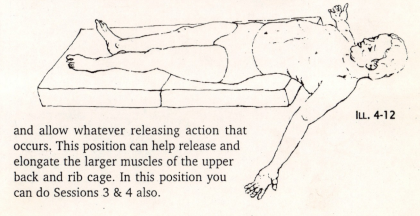

ILL. 4-12

and allow whatever releasing action that
occurs. This position can help release and
elongate the larger muscles of the upper
back and rib cage. In this position you
can do Sessions 3 & 4 also.

49

Session 6

In this variation of session 5 there will be no particular movement required other than breathing comfortably for a long period of time. This position, because of its low impact can be done for very long periods of time with very good results, since it puts your body in a position that is open and expanded. See **Ill. 4-12**. This helps reverse some of the habits or tendencies to close or collapse your body. This is a very good position to recover from a strenuous day. Many clients say they will listen to music, talk with friends, or watch TV in this position. When you have lain in this position for an hour or more, the releases are very definite.

Take the very same position as #5 with pillows supporting your lower back and legs. Your shoulders and head are resting on the ground. Place your arms out to the sides with your palms facing up. Start a comfortable breathing pattern that is full and has the feeling of reaching all areas of your body. You can do this for a period of 1/2 hour or more. You set the time that feels comfortable to you.

This chapter of Alignment Releasing Sessions gives you a variety of techniques that you can use for initially releasing the body and later as a means of relaxing and maintaining the releases that you have had. The sessions are easy to do and you will always find them useful.

Summary

The subjects of breathing and alignment are tools that will serve you through life. The application of breathing whether it's one big breath or many breaths is a daily function you can become more mindful of for relaxation and maintaining your alignment. The awareness of breathing is also a perfect centering process for you to utilize during the day.

You can give yourself a breathing session anywhere at any time without interfering with the chores at hand. At first it may be a discipline that you set for your self, then it becomes a way of having an awareness of your body in time and space.

If you have physical problems you may be able to find ways to relieve or release them by creating space in the afflicted areas and applying a releasing session for that area of the body. However, if the problem does persist, it is advisable that you seek professional consultation.

For the professional athlete or performer there are many areas of exploration where breathing and the knowledge of alignment can give you insights into the efficiency and mastery of the particular skills involved with your field.

All in all, you have the tools to embark on a journey of physical understanding that can extend into every area of your life. Good luck and blessings.

Harmon Hathaway

INDEX

NEW AGE BOOKS

TIBETAN POWER YOGA—*Jutta Mattausch*
This is one of the oldest exercises in the world. The "Tibetan Power Yoga" is what the Tibetan Lama Tsering Norbu calls a set of motions that has given the people from the Roof of the World, physical vitality and mental power up into ripe old age since time immemorial.
ISBN: 81-7822-006-7

ENERGETIC HEALING—*Arnie Lade*
Embracing the Life Force is a guide to the inner landscape of subtle energy. In this groundbreaking book the role, manifestation, utility and healing power of our life force/energy is explored in a concise and informative fashion.
ISBN: 81-7822-005-9

MAGNETIC HEALING—*Buryl Payne*
Discover the positive benefits of magnetism for improving your health and well being.
❑ What ailments can be treated with magnets?
❑ How do magnets work to heal the body?
❑ What is the correct way to use magnets?
Find the answers to these questions and more!
ISBN: 81-7822-002-4

CHAKRA ENERGY MASSAGE—*Marianne Uhl*
This book guides you into the fascinating world of the energy body. Drawing on the knowledge gained by Foot Reflexology Massage, it introduces you to the Chakra Energy Massage. She provides detailed information on the healing effects of gemstones and the powers of fragrant essences, as well as the vibrations of primal tones and various colours, all of which can be employed to effectively enhance your work with the Chakras.
ISBN: 81-7822-004-0

PENDULUM HEALING HANDBOOK—*Walter Lübeck*
If you want to learn every aspect of how to use a pendulum, particularly in relation to methods of alternative healing, this book is for you. It answers the questions that normally occur following a person's first experiences with the pendulum.
ISBN: 81-7822-003-2

NAB 39

UNDERSTANDING YOUR BODY ALIGNMENT
—Harmon Hathaway
The book offers very effective techniques for releasing tension and frozen energy, helping the body to function freely, as it was meant to function.
ISBN: 81-7822-001-6

STRESS-FREE WORK WITH YOGA AND AYURVEDA
—Vinod Verma
Dr. Verma's advice for a stress-free work environment begins with a daily yoga program—easy exercises that take a total of sixteen minutes a day! She shows you how to recognize the three basic Ayurvedic types so you can "read" the people you work with.
ISBN: 81-7822-000-8

THE INTUITIVE WAY—Penney Peirce
There's never been a book like The Intuitive Way! Comprehensive, easy, and entertaining to read, the author's no-nonsense approach inspires and instructs as no previous book on intuitive development has ever done.

QUANTUM-TOUCH THE POWER TO HEAL—Richard Gordon
Quantum-Touch represents a major breakthrough in the art of hands-on healing. Whether you are a complete novice, a professional chiropractor, physical therapist, body worker, healer, or other health professional, Quantum-Touch allows you a dimension of power in your work that heretofore has not seemed possible. Since the body already knows how to heal itself, the practitioner need only apply the energy to affected areas.

THE TANTRIC PATH TO HIGHER CONSCIOUSNESS
—Sunyata Saraswati, Bodhi Avinasha
At last these ancient secrets are emerging from the monasteries and mystery schools. Some of the most powerful techniques ever devised by man to accelerate his evolution are now yours to use. Now you can learn to direct the life force in your body, the creative sexual power. You can increase your energy level, heal and rejuvenate yourself, enjoy the psychic sensitivity which develops spontaneously in this practice.